Slow Co

Slow Cooker Recipes For Beginners

(Slow Cooker Recipe That Will Help You Loose Weigh)

Rodney Williamsons

Table Of Contents

Slow Cooker Shrimp and Artichoke Barley Risotto

Ingredients:

- 2 cups pearl barley
- 4 oz parmesan cheese, grated
- 8 oz baby spinach
- 6 tsp Better that Bouillon Lobster Base
- 6 cloves garlic, mined
- 2 lb shrimp, peeled deveined
- 4 tsp grated lemon zest
- Freshly ground black pepper to taste
- Salt to taste
- 2 Tbsp olive oil
- 6 cups water
- 2 chopped cups onions

- 2 packages frozen artichoke hearts, thawed, quartered

Instructions:

1. Place a saucepan with 6 cups water over high heat. Bring to a boil.
2. Turn off the heat.
3. Add lobster base to boiling water.
4. Whisk well and keep it aside.
5. Place a nonstick skillet over medium-low heat.
6. Add oil and heat.
7. When oil is heated, add onions and sauté until translucent.
8. Add garlic and sauté until aromatic.
9. Transfer into the slow cooker.
10. Add lobster base solution and rest of the ingredients except

spinach, lemon zest, cheese, and shrimp.

11.   Cover and cook for 6 hours on low or for 4 hours on high or until barley is tender and liquid in the pot is dry.

12.   Add shrimp and cheese and stir.

13.   Cover and cook for 2 0-35 minutes or until shrimp turn opaque.

14.   Add lemon zest and baby spinach.

15.   Mix well. Taste and adjust the seasoning if required.

16.   Cover and let it sit for 6 minutes or until spinach wilts.

i. Serve hot.

Shrimp and Grits

Ingredients:
- Kosher salt to taste
- 8 cups vegetable stock
- 2 cups whole milk
- 2 cups frozen corn kernels
- Red hot pepper sauce, to taste
- 2 lb shrimp
- 4 cups corn grits, stone ground
- 2 cups heavy whipping cream
- 2 cup diced cheese
- 2 jalapeño peppers, diced

Instructions:
1. Add grits, cream, vegetable broth, cheese, hot sauce, milk, corn, jalapeño pepper and salt into the slow cooker and mix well.

2. Cover and cook for 4 -4 hours on low or until cooked.
3. Add more broth if required.
4. Stir occasionally.
5. Stir in the shrimp and cover again.
6. Cook until shrimp turns opaque.
7. Serve in bowls.

Moroccan-Spiced Slow-Cooked Fish

Ingredients:
- 8 cloves garlic, minced
- 4 Tbsp olive oil
- 2 tsp cumin
- 2 tsp ground coriander
- 1 tsp cayenne pepper
- 1 cup chopped cilantro + extra to garnish
- 4 tbsp fresh lemon juice
- 2 Tbsp paprika
- 4 tsp kosher salt
- 1 teaspoon ground turmeric
- 4 lb halibut steaks or halibut /cod/salmon fillets

Instructions:

1. Add garlic, oil, cumin, coriander, cayenne pepper, cilantro, lemon juice, paprika, salt and turmeric into a Ziploc bag.
2. Close the bag and shake until well combined.
3. Add fish into the bag.
4. Close it and shake the bag so that the fish is well coated with the marinade.
5. Chill for 6 -6 hours.
6. Add 1/2 cup water into the slow cooker.
7. Transfer the contents of the bag into the slow cooker.
8. Cover and cook for 4 -2 hours or until the fish flakes easily when pierced with a fork.
9. When done, uncover and let it rest for 6 minutes.
10. Garnish with cilantro and serve.

Basic Lamb Roast

Ingredients:

- 2 1 Tbsp cumin
- 2 1 tsp garlic powder
- 2 1 tsp chili powder
- 4 lb lamb roast
- 24 oz diced green chilies
- 25 oz fire roasted diced tomatoes
- 2 red bell peppers, diced
- 2 green bell pepper, diced
- 2 1 Tbsp paprika

    Salt
- Black pepper
- Nonstick cooking spray

Instructions:

1. Place a heavy bottomed skillet over medium flame and grease with non-stick cooking spray.

2. Brown the lamb roast all over.

3. Place the browned lamb roast into the slow cooker and add the bell pepper, tomatoes and chilies.

4. Stir in the paprika, cumin, chili and garlic powders, then season with salt and pepper.

5. Pour just enough water to cover the bottom of the slow cooker.

6. Cover and cook on low for 8 hours, adding more water if needed.

7. Take the lamb out of the slow cooker and shred using a fork.

8. Pour the sauce all over it and serve warm.

Apple Mustard Pork Belly

Ingredients:

- 6 Tbsp Italian seasoning
- 2 1 Tbsp salt
- 4 Tbsp Dijon or whole grain mustard
- 4 lb pork belly, sliced into chunks
- 6 medium apples, peeled, cored, and sliced into chunks

Instructions:

1. Combine the salt, Italian seasoning and mustard in the slow cooker.

2. Add the pork belly and toss to coat.

3. Toss in the apples until evenly distributed, then cover and cook on low heat for 8 hours or until pork belly is cooked through. Serve hot.

11

Chipotle Beef

Ingredients:
- 2 lb beef tenderloin, cubed
- 1 cup beef stock
- 2 Tbsp chopped chipotle chili
- 1/2 cup mild gluten free salsa

Salt
- Black pepper

Instructions:

1. Combine the beef tenderloin, stock, chipotle chili and salsa in the slow cooker.

2. Cover and cook for 6 hours on low. Season to taste with salt and pepper.

Poultry and Seafood

Ingredients:

- 2 tsp chili powder
- 1/2 tsp ground cinnamon
- 1 tsp salt
- 1 Tbsp Mexican herb and spice blend paste
- 2 banana
- 2 sweet tart apple
- 2 Tbsp almond flour
- 2 Tbsp olive oil
- 25 /4 lbs skinless, boneless chicken thighs
- 1 cup chopped sweet onions
- 1 cup diced green bell peppers
- 2 /8 cup slivered almonds
- 1/2 cup crushed tomatoes

- 8 1 ounces canned mandarin orange segments, drained with juices reserved

Instructions:

1. Heat the oil in a skillet over medium flame.

2. Brown the chicken for 5 minute on both sides, then transfer to a 4 -quart slow cooker.

3. Saute the onions, bell peppers and almonds for 4 minutes then transfer the mixture into a blender and add the crushed tomatoes, 1/2 cup of the reserved mandarin orange juice, salt, chili powder, cinnamon, and Mexican herb and spice blend paste.

4. Puree to a smooth consistency.

5. Pour the mixture on top of the chicken in the slow cooker.

6. Cover and cook for 4 hours on low.

7. In the meantime, peel the apple and banana.

8. Core and slice the apple, and slice the banana into 1 inch pieces.

9. Add the banana and apple along with the mandarin oranges into the slow cooker.

10. Cover and cook for an additional hour or until the apples become fork tender.

11. Using a slotted spoon, transfer the chicken and fruit to a serving platter and cover with aluminum foil to keep warm.

12. Put the almond flour in a bowl and stir in 1 cup of the sauce from the slow cooker.

13. Pour the mixture back into the slow cooker, cover and cook for 6 minutes on high, or until the sauce becomes thick.

14.   Pour the sauce on top of the fruit and chicken then serve immediately.

Indian Chicken and Cashew Stew

Ingredients:

- 2 chickens, 4 lb each, chopped into serving pieces
- 2 cups cashew nuts, divided
- 4 cups chicken stock
- 6 Tbsp vegetable oil
- 2 carrots, diced
- 2 large onions, diced
- Sea salt
- Freshly ground black pepper
- 25 oz chilled coconut cream
- 8 garlic cloves, minced
- 4 Tbsp curry powder
- 4 Tbsp grated fresh ginger

- 1 tsp cayenne
- 2 tsp ground cinnamon

Instructions:

1. In a large resealable plastic bag, mix together the coconut cream, garlic, ginger, cinnamon, curry powder, and cayenne.

2. Season with salt and pepper to taste.

3. Rinse the chicken pieces, then pat dry using paper towels.

4. Place inside the plastic bag with the marinade.

5. Seal and turn several times to coat.

6. Refrigerate for 6 to 25 hours, turning occasionally.

7. Preheat the broiler and line a broiler pan using aluminum foil.

8. Broil the chicken until browned, for about 4 minutes per side.

9. Combine 2 cup stock and 2 1 cups cashew nuts in a food processor.

10.   Grind to a paste.

11.   Add remaining cashews and pulse coarsely. Set aside.

12.   Heat a skillet over medium high flame and add the oil.

13.   Saute the onion until translucent. Add the carrot, cashew nut mixture, and remaining stock.

14.   Add the marinade.

15.   Mix everything thoroughly, then bring to a boil and transfer to the slow cooker.

16.   Add the chicken into the slow cooker, skin sides facing down.

17.   Cover and cook for 8 hours on low or for 4 hours on high, or until chicken is completely cooked.

18.   Season with salt and pepper to taste, then serve.

Tarragon and Mustard Chicken Stew

Ingredients:

- 2 small celery rib, chopped
- 2 Tbsp Dijon mustard
- 2 tsp dried tarragon leaves
- 2 tsp molasses
- 1 tsp lemon juice
- 2 Tbsp almond flour
- 2 /8 cup water
- 1 lb boneless, skinless chicken breast, cubed
- 1 cup chopped onion
- 1 cup sliced carrots
- 1 cup small Brussels sprouts

- 1 cup low sodium fat free chicken broth

Instructions:

1. Mix the chicken, broth, fresh onion, carrots, Brussels sprouts, celery, mustard, tarragon, molasses and lemon juice in the slow cooker. Stir well.

2. Cover the slow cooker and cook for 6 hours on low.

3. After that, increase the heat to high and cook for additional 25 minutes.

4. Mix together the water and almond flour, then stir this into the stew for 1 to 5 minutes .

5. Season with salt and pepper to taste and serve over hot cauliflower rice.

Springtime Vegetable and Chicken

Ingredients:

- 6 Tbsp chopped fresh parsley
- 4 garlic cloves, minced
- 25 oz frozen pearl onions, thawed
- 25 oz frozen peas, thawed
- 4 heads Bibb lettuce, trimmed and quartered
- Sea salt
- Freshly ground black pepper
- 2 chickens, 4 lbs each, chopped into serving pieces
- 4 cups chicken stock
- 2 Tbsp fresh chopped rosemary or 2 tsp dried
- 2 Tbsp fresh thyme or 2 tsp dried
- 2 Tbsp fresh tarragon or 2 tsp dried
- 2 bay leaves

Instructions:

1. Rinse the chicken and pat dry using paper towels.

2. Preheat the broiler and line a broiler pan with aluminum foil.

3. Broil the chicken until browned, for about 4 minutes per side.

4. Combine the thyme, parsley, tarragon, bay leaves, rosemary, garlic, pearl onions, and stock in the slow cooker.

5. Place the chicken pieces on top, skin side facing down.

6. Cover and cook for 8 hours on low or for 4 hours and 45 minutes on high, or until chicken is completely cooked.

7. Set heat to high, then add the lettuce and peas. Cover and cook for 40 minutes, or until chicken is very tender.

8. Take out the bay leaves, then season with salt and pepper to taste. Serve warm.

Chicken Gumbo

Ingredients:

- 1 cup chopped onion
- 1/2 cup chopped green or red bell pepper
- 1/2 tsp dried thyme leaves
- 2 garlic clove, minced
- 2 /8 tsp crushed red pepper
- 4 ounces fresh or frozen and thawed small okra, cut in half
- 1 lb chicken breast, cut into 1/3 inch cubes
- 8 1 ounces stewed tomatoes
- 2 cup low sodium fat free chicken broth

Instructions:

1. Mix the chicken, tomatoes, broth, fresh onion, bell pepper, garlic, thyme, and crushed red pepper in the slow cooker.

2. Cover and cook for 6 hours on low, stirring in the okra within the last half hour.

3. Season with salt and pepper to taste and serve on top of hot cauliflower rice.

Sweet and Sour Caribbean Chicken

Ingredients:

- 2 cup dark rum
- 2 cup cider vinegar
- 2 cup raw honey or high quality maple syrup
- 4 Tbsp almond flour
- Sea salt
- Freshly ground black pepper
- 2 chickens, 4 lb each, chopped into serving pieces
- 4 large onions, sliced thinly
- 6 garlic cloves, minced
- 6 Tbsp olive oil
- 6 Tbsp grated fresh ginger
- 4 cups chicken stock

Instructions:

1. Rinse the chicken, then pat dry using paper towels.

2. Preheat the broiler and line a broiler pan using aluminum foil.

3. Broil the chicken until browned, about 4 minutes per side.

4. Heat the oil over medium high flame in a skillet.

5. Sauté the fresh onion, ginger, and garlic until onion is translucent.

6. Transfer to the slow cooker.

7. Add the vinegar, stock, raw honey or maple syrup, and rum.

8. Combine thoroughly.

9. Place the chicken pieces inside the slow cooker with the skin facing down.

10.　　　Cover and cook for 8 hours on low or for 4 hours on high, or until the chicken is cooked through.

11.　　　Set heat to high. Mix together the almond flour and 4 tablespoons of water in a bowl, then stir into the slow cooker.

12.　　　Cook for 25 minutes, or until simmering and thickened.

13.　　　Season with salt and pepper to taste, then serve.

Italian-Style Fish Stew

Ingredients:

- 1/3 lb tomatoes, peeled and chopped
- 2 small garlic cloves, minced
- 1 cup halved small mushrooms
- 2 tsp dried Italian seasoning
- 2 /8 tsp crushed red pepper
- 1 lb firm fleshed fish steaks such as grouper, sliced thinly
- 1/2 cup chopped parsley
- 1 cup low sodium fat free chicken broth or clam juice
- 1/2 cup dry white wine or chicken broth

Instructions:

1. Stir together the broth or clam juice, wine or broth, tomatoes, mushrooms,

31

garlic, Italian seasoning, and red pepper in the slow cooker.

2. Cover and cook for 4 hours on high.

3. Add the parsley and fish 25 minutes before the end of cooking time.

4. Season with salt and pepper to taste, stir, and serve.

Moroccan Fish Stew

Ingredients:

- 2 tsp ground ginger
- 2 tsp ground cumin
- 2 Tbsp paprika
- 2 cups seafood stock
- 2 cup sliced pimiento stuffed green olives
- 4 bay leaves
- Sea salt
- Cayenne pepper
- Freshly ground black pepper
- 4 lb halibut, cod, or other firm white fish fillet, sliced into 8 pieces
- 2 1 cups olive oil, divided
- 1 cup dry white wine
- 1 cup freshly squeezed lemon juice
- 4 Tbsp chopped fresh cilantro
- 4 large onions, diced

- 6 garlic cloves, minced

Instructions:

1. Rinse the fish fillets and pat dry, then set aside.

2. In a bowl, combine 2 cup olive oil with the wine, lemon juice, paprika, cilantro, cumin, and ginger.

3. Add salt and cayenne pepper to taste. Pour mixture into a resealable plastic bag.

4. Add the fish fillets into the marinade, then seal the bag and refrigerate for at least 4 hours, turning occasionally.

5. Heat the rest of the olive oil in a skillet over medium high flame.

6. Sauté the onion and garlic until onion is translucent.

7. Transfer to the slow cooker.

8. Drain the marinade from the plastic bag and add to the slow cooker.

9. Place fish bag into the refrigerator.

10.   Add the olives, stock, and bay leaves into the slow cooker.

11.   Combine thoroughly.

12.   Cover and cook for 6 hours on low or for 4 hours on high.

13.   Set heat to high and add the fish.

14.   Cover and cook for 40 minutes, or until fish is cooked through.

15.   Take out the bay leaves, then season with salt and pepper to taste. Serve at once.

Chocolate And Liquor Cream

Ingredients:

- ounces dark chocolate, cut into chunks2 teaspoon liquor
- 2 teaspoon sugar
- ounces crème fraiche

Directions:

1. In your slow cooker,
2. mix crème fraiche with chocolate, liquor and sugar,
3. stir, cover,
4. cook on Low for 2 hours,
5. divide into bowls and serve cold

Dates And Rice Pudding

Ingredients:

- 2 cup almond milk
- tablespoons brown sugar
- 2 teaspoon almond extract
- 2 cup dates, chopped
- 1 cup white rice

Directions:

1. In your slow cooker, mix the rice with the milk and the other ingredients, whisk, put the lid on and cook on Low for 4 hours.
2. Divide the pudding into bowls and serve.

Butternut Squash Sweet Mix

Ingredients:

- 2 cup milk - ¾ cup maple syrup
- 2 teaspoon cinnamon powder
- 1 teaspoon ginger powder
- 1/2 teaspoon cloves, ground
- 2 tablespoon cornstarch
- Whipped cream for serving
- pounds butternut squash, steamed, peeled and mashed
- fresh eggs

Directions:

1. In a bowl, mix squash with maple syrup, milk, fresh eggs, cinnamon, cornstarch, ginger, cloves and cloves and stir very well.
2. Pour this into your slow cooker, cover, cook on Low for 2 hours,

divide into cups and serve with whipped cream on top.

Almonds, Walnuts And Mango Bowls

Ingredients:
- 2 cup heavy cream
- 1 teaspoon vanilla extract
- 2 teaspoon almond extract
- 2 tablespoon brown sugar
- 2 cup walnuts, chopped
- tablespoons almonds, chopped
- 2 cup mango, peeled and roughly cubed

Directions:
1. In your slow cooker, mix the nuts with the mango, cream and the other

ingredients, toss, put the lid on and cook on High for 2 hours.
2. Divide the mix into bowls and serve.

Tapioca Pudding

Ingredients:

- 1 cup water
- 1 cup sugar
- Zest of 1 fresh lemon
- 2 and 1/2 cups milk
- 1/2 cup tapioca pearls, rinsed

Directions:

1. In your slow cooker, mix tapioca with milk, sugar, water and fresh lemon zest, stir, cover, cook on Low for 2 hour, divide into cups and serve warm.

Berries Salad

Ingredients:

- 1 cup cranberries
- 2 cup blackberries
- 2 cup strawberries
- 1 cup heavy cream
- tablespoons brown sugar
- 2 tablespoon lime juice
- 2 tablespoon lime zest, grated
- 2 cup blueberries

Directions:

2. In your slow cooker, mix the berries with the sugar and the other ingredients, toss, put the lid on and cook on High for 2 hour.
3. Divide the mix into bowls and serve.

Paprika Peppers

Ingredients:

- 2 teaspoon salt
- 2 spring onions, chopped
- 1 teaspoon ground black pepper
- 1 cup of coconut milk
- 2 cup red bell peppers, cut into strips
- 2 cup green bell peppers, cut into strips
- 2 teaspoon keto tomato sauce
- 2 teaspoon hot paprika

Directions:

1. In the slow cooker, mix the peppers with the paprika and the other ingredients and close the lid.
2. Cook the peppers for 4 hours on Low.

Savoury Almond Bread

Ingredients:

- 1/2 cup basil pesto sauce
- 1/2 cup Parmesan
- 4 Cheddar cheese, grated
- 2 cup coconut milk
- 2 cups ground almonds
- 1 cup flax seed meal
- Salt and pepper to taste
- 1 teaspoon baking soda
- 2 large eggs

Directions:

1. Combine dry ingredients in a bowl.
2. Blend wet ingredients in another bowl.
3. Mix the two slowly.
4. Butter the crock-pot, pour in the batter.
5. Cover the crock-pot with a paper towel to absorb the water.
6. Cover, cook on low for 4 hours.

Chocolate Walnut Pie

Ingredients:

- 2 tablespoon chocolate chips, melted
- 1/2 cup peanut butter
- 2 tablespoon Erythritol
- 1 cup coconut flakes
- 2 cup of coconut milk
- 4 cup almond flour
- 2 teaspoon almond extract
- 4 tablespoons walnuts chopped

Directions:

1. Mix up together coconut milk with the flour and the other ingredients and stir.
2. When the mixture is homogenous, pour it in the crockpot.
3. Add butter and close the lid.
4. Cook the mix for 2.6 hours.

Fruity Custard Delight

Ingredients:
- 1/2 teaspoon of cinnamon, ground
- To serve:
- 2 cup of whipped cream
- 2 lb. keto sponge cake, sliced
- Mix berries, sliced
- 6 eggs
- 1/3 cup of brown swerve
- 2 teaspoon of vanilla extract
- 2 pinch salt

Directions:
1. Start by blending all the Ingredients: together in a mixer.
2. Pour this mixture into a steel pan and place it in the Crockpot.
3. Cover its lid and cook for 4 hours on Low setting.
4. Once done, remove its lid of the crockpot carefully.
5. Allow it to cool and refrigerate for 2 hour.

6. To serve, layer a casserole dish with sponge cake slices.
7. Top them with prepared custard and garnish with fresh fruits.
8. Refrigerate again for 4 hours or more.
9. Serve.

Lemon Cheese Cake

Ingredients:

- 1 tablespoon of Lemon Juice
- zest of half lemon
- 4 egg, room temp
- 1 jar lemon curd
- 4 raspberries
- 2 cup of water
- 1/2 cup of erythritol
- 1 teaspoon of almond flour
- 1/2 teaspoon of vanilla
- 2 tablespoons of sour cream

Directions:

1. Separately blend the wet and dry Ingredients: in the mixer while reserving the berries
2. Mix both the mixtures together in a bowl until smooth.
3. Now spread the cake batter in a greased ramekin and place it in the Crockpot.

4. Cover its lid and cook for 6 hours on Low setting.
5. Once done, remove its lid of the crockpot carefully.
6. Allow it to cool and refrigerate for 2 hour.
7. Garnish with the berries
8. Serve.

Keto Fudge

Ingredients:
- 1 cup Erythritol
- 2 teaspoon vanilla extract
- 4 tablespoons cocoa powder
- 2 tablespoon cream cheese
- 6 tablespoons butter
- 2 oz dark chocolate
- 4 tablespoons almond flour

Directions:
1. Combine the butter and dark chocolate and preheat the mixture.
2. When the mixture is melted, add the almond flour, Erythritol, vanilla extract, and cocoa powder.
3. Add the cream cheese and stir.
4. Place the fudge mixture in the slow cooker and cook it for 4 hours on High.
5. Serve the cooked fudge hot!

Cashew Cream Mix

Ingredients:

- 1 cup coconut cream
- 2 tablespoons allulose
- ¾ teaspoon baking soda
- 1 teaspoon vanilla extract
- 2 cup cashew milk
- ¾ cup cashew butter

Directions:

1. In the crockpot, mix the cashew with cashew butter and the other ingredients and close the lid.
2. Cook on Low for 8 .6 hours.
3. Stir the cooked meal well and pour in the glass jar.

Almond Cookies

Ingredients:

- 2 teaspoon vanilla extract
- 2 teaspoon baking powder
- 2 tablespoons Erythritol
- 2 oz almonds, chopped
- 4 tablespoons butter
- 1 cup almond flour

Directions:

1. Combine the almond flour, vanilla extract, baking powder, and Erythritol.
2. Stir the mixture and add butter.
3. Knead into a smooth dough.
4. Make fresh balls from the dough and sprinkle the balls with the almonds.
5. Press the almond into the cookies gently.
6. Transfer the cookies to the slow cooker.
7. Cook the cookies for 2 hours on High.
8. Cool the cookies.
9. Enjoy!

Keto Flan

Ingredients:

- 1 teaspoon vanilla extract
- 1/2 cup Swerve
- 1 teaspoon butter
- 1 cup water, for cooking
- 2 cup heavy cream
- 4 eggs, beaten

Directions:

1. Put butter in the skillet and melt it.
2. Add Swerve and simmer the liquid over the fresh heat for 4 minutes.
3. Then pour the butter sweet mixture into the ramekins.
4. Mix up together beaten eggs, vanilla extract, and heavy cream.
5. When the liquid is smooth, pour it over the sweet butter mixture in the ramekins.
6. Pour water in the crockpot.

7. Place the ramekins with flan in the water and close the lid.
8. Cook flan for 25 hours on Low.
9. Chill the flan little and turn the ramekins over in the plates to get flan.

Almond Cheese Cake

Ingredients:

- 2 tablespoon of powdered peanut butter
- 1 teaspoon of pure vanilla extract
- 1/2 cup of almonds, sliced
- 2 egg
- 8oz. cream cheese softened

Directions:

1. Separately blend the wet and dry Ingredients: in the mixer while reserving the berries.
2. Mix both the mixtures together in a bowl until smooth.
3. Now spread the cake batter in a greased ramekin and place it in the Crockpot.
4. Cover its lid and cook for 3-4 hours on Low setting.
5. Once done, remove its lid of the crockpot carefully.
6. Allow it to cool and refrigerate for 2 hour.
7. Serve.

Cinnamon Cup Cake

Ingredients:

- 1 cup coconut flour
- 1 teaspoon baking soda
- 2 tablespoon stevia extract
- 2 oz walnuts, chopped
- 2 teaspoon ground cinnamon
- 2 eggs
- 2 cup almond milk, unsweetened

Directions:

1. Beat the eggs in a big bowl and whisk well.
2. Add ground cinnamon and almond milk and stir gently.
3. Then add baking soda and stevia extract.
4. Whisk the mixture until smooth and add chopped walnuts.
5. Stir the batter and place it in fresh ramekins.
6. Put the ramekins in the slow cooker and cook for 4 hours on High.

7. Serve the dessert immediately!

Pecan Pie

Ingredients:

- 2 tablespoon lemon juice
- 2 cups almond flour
- 4 tablespoons Erythritol
- 2 teaspoon vanilla extract
- 2 tablespoon chocolate chips
- 4 tablespoons peanut butter
- 4 pecans, chopped
- 2 teaspoon baking powder

Directions:

1. Make the dough: in the mixing bowl, mix up together chocolate chips, peanut butter, chopped pecans, baking powder, lemon juice, almond flour, Erythritol, and vanilla extract.
2. Knead the smooth and non-sticky dough.
3. Then line the crockpot with baking paper.

4. Make the shape of bun from the dough and put it in the crockpot.
5. Flatten it well with the help of the fingertips.
6. Close the lid and cook pecan pie for 4 .6 hours on High.
7. Chill the cooked pie well and then remove from the crockpot.
8. Slice it into the servings.

Vanilla Cake

Ingredients:
- 2 teaspoon apple cider vinegar
- 2 tablespoons Erythritol
- 2 teaspoons vanilla extract
- 4 eggs, beaten
- 4 tablespoons chocolate chips, softened
- 2 cup organic coconut milk
- 2 cup almond flour
- 2 teaspoon baking powder

Directions:
1. In the big bowl combine together the coconut milk with the flour and the other ingredients and whisk.
2. Line the slow cooker with the baking paper.
3. Pour the batter in the slow cooker.
4. Flatten it with the help of the spatula if needed.
5. Cook the cake for 6 hours on Low.

6. Then chill the cake well and remove it from the slow cooker.
7. Discard the baking paper and cut the cake into the servings.

Walnut Squares

Ingredients:

- 1 cup coconut flour
- 2 teaspoon baking soda
- 2 tablespoon butter, softened
- Cooking spray
- 2 cup walnuts, chopped
- 2 tablespoons stevia
- 2 teaspoon vanilla extract
- 2 eggs, beaten
- 2 cup

Directions:

1. Spray the crockpot with cooking spray from inside.
2. In the mixing bowl, combine the walnuts with stevia and the other ingredients and stir until you obtain a dough.
3. Transfer the dough in the crockpot and flatten it well with the help of the spatula.
4. Close the lid and cook the dough for 4 hours on High.

5. The time of cooking depends on the dough thicknesses.
6. When the dough is cooked, carefully transfer it on the chopping board and let chill to the room temperature.
7. Cut it into the squares.

Raspberry Cake

Ingredients:

- 6 tablespoons of Organic Valley Pasture Butter melted
- 2/4 cup of water
- 1 teaspoon of vanilla extract
- Filling
- 8 oz. Organic Valley cream cheese
- 1/2 cup of erythritol
- 2 large egg
- 2 tablespoons of Organic Valley whipping cream
- 5 cup of fresh raspberries
- 2 1/2 almond flour
- 1 cup of Swerve
- 1/2 cup of coconut flour
- 1/2 cup of Organic Valley Vanilla Fuel Protein Powder
- 5 teaspoons of baking powder
- 1/2 teaspoon of salt
- 4 large eggs

Directions:

1. Separately blend the cake mixture and the filling in the mixer while reserving the berries.
2. Now spread the cake batter in the greased based on your crockpot.
3. Top it with the prepared filling evenly and spread the berries over it.
4. Cover its lid and cook for 4 hours on Low setting.
5. Once done, remove its lid of the crockpot carefully.
6. Allow it to cool and refrigerate for 2 hour.
7. Serve.

Carrot Walnut Cake

Ingredients:

- 1/3 teaspoons of apple pie spice
- 2 tablespoons of coconut oil
- 1/2 cup of heavy whipping cream
- 1 cup of carrots shredded
- 1/2 cup of walnuts diced
- 1 cup of almond flour
- 1/2 cup of Brown swerve
- 1 teaspoon of baking powder

Directions:

1. Separately blend the wet and dry Ingredients: in the mixer.
2. Mix both the mixtures together in a bowl until smooth.
3. Now spread the cake batter in a greased ramekin and place it in the Crockpot.
4. Cover its lid and cook for 6 hours on Low setting.
5. Once done, remove its lid of the crockpot carefully.

6. Allow it to cool and refrigerate for 2 hour.
7. Serve.

Granola

Ingredients:
- 2 cup of sunflower seeds
- 2 cup of pumpkin seeds
- 2 cup of shredded coconut
- 1 cup of Swerve
- 2 teaspoon of cinnamon, ground
- 2 teaspoon of salt
- 2 cup of whipped cream
- 2 teaspoon of vanilla extract
- 1 cup of raw almonds
- 1 cup of walnuts
- 1 cup of pecans
- 1 cup of hazelnuts

Directions:
1. Start by putting everything in the Crockpot and mix well.
2. Cover its lid and cook for 2 hours on Low setting.
3. Once done, remove its lid of the crockpot carefully.

4. Spread the mixture on a baking sheet and leave for 45 minutes.
5. Slice and serve.

Lavender Crème Brule

Ingredients:

- 2 tablespoon of vanilla extract
- 1 cup of swerve
- 1 tablespoon of lavender buds
- 6 egg yolks
- 2 cups of heavy cream

Directions:

1. Start by blending all the Ingredients: except lavender in a blender until smooth.
2. Now divide the batter into 4 ramekins and place them in the Crockpot.
3. Cover its lid and cook for 2 hours on Low setting.
4. Once done, remove its lid of the crockpot carefully.
5. Allow it to cool and refrigerate for 2 hour.
6. Garnish with lavender.
7. Serve.

Walnut Muffins

Ingredients:

- 2 egg
- 2 tablespoons liquid stevia
- 4 tablespoons almond milk, unsweetened
- 2 teaspoon baking powder
- 2 oz walnuts, chopped
- 6 tablespoons butter
- 2 cup coconut flour
- 2 teaspoon vanilla extract

Directions:

1. Mix the butter, flour, vanilla extract, liquid stevia, almond milk, and baking powder.
2. Beat the egg into the mixture and whisk it well until smooth.
3. Add the chopped walnuts and stir well.
4. Place the dough in the muffin molds and transfer into the slow cooker.
5. Cook the muffins for 4 hours on High.
6. Cool the cooked muffins and enjoy!

Chocolate Cream Custard

Ingredients:
- 1/2 teaspoon of cinnamon, ground
- Sugar-free chocolate, grated
- Whipped cream
- 6 eggs
- 1/3 cup of brown swerve
- 2 teaspoon of vanilla extract
- 2 teaspoon of cocoa powder

Directions:
1. Start by blending all the Ingredients: together in a mixer.
2. Pour this mixture into 4 ramekins and place them in the Crockpot.
3. Cover its lid and cook for 2 hours on Low setting.
4. Once done, remove its lid of the crockpot carefully.
5. Allow it to cool and refrigerate for 2 hour.

6. Garnish with chocolate and whipped cream.
7. Serve.

Zucchini Cake

Ingredients:
- 2 zucchinis, grated
- 2 tablespoons pecans, chopped
- 1/2 cup organic coconut milk
- 2 eggs, beaten
- 1/2 cup stevia
- 2 teaspoon coconut oil
- 2 tablespoons cream cheese
- 2 cup almond flour
- 4 tablespoons coconut flour
- 2 teaspoon baking soda
- 1 teaspoon apple cider vinegar
- 2 teaspoon cocoa powder

Directions:
1. In the mixing bowl mix up together the flour with the baking soda and the other ingredients and whisk.
2. Line the slow cooker with baking paper and transfer the cake mixture inside.
3. Flatten it gently.

4. Cook the cake for 4 hours on Low.
5. Cut the cake into the servings.

Chocolate Muffins

Ingredients:

- 1 teaspoon ground cinnamon
- 2 cup almond flour
- 4 teaspoons stevia
- 2 egg, beaten
- 2 tablespoon chocolate chips, softened
- 1 cup butter, softened
- 2 teaspoon baking soda

Directions:

1. Make the muffin batter: in a bowl, mix the chocolate with the butter and the other ingredients and whisk.
2. Pour it in the muffin molds and transfer in the crockpot.
3. Cook the muffins for 2.6 hours on High.

Slim Waist, Rich Taste Chocolate Cake

Ingredients:
- 2 teaspoons baking powder
- 1/2 teaspoon salt
- 1 cup butter, melted 4 large eggs
- ¾ unsweetened almond milk
- 2 teaspoon vanilla extract
- 4 cups almond flour
- ¾ cup granulated or powdered sweetener of your choice
- ⅔ cup cocoa powder
- 1/2 cup whey protein powder

Directions:
1. In a bowl, mix the dry ingredients.
2. Stir in the wet ingredients one at a time.
3. Combine thoroughly.
4. Butter the crock-pot. Pour in the cake batter.
5. Cover, cook on low for 4 hours.

6. Switch off. Let it set uncovered for 45 minutes.

Blackberry Pancake

Ingredients:

- 4 eggs, beaten
- 2 tablespoon stevia
- 2 teaspoon butter
- 1/2 cup coconut cream
- Cooking spray
- 2 cup almond flour
- 1 cup coconut flour
- 2 teaspoon vanilla extract
- 1/2 teaspoon ground nutmeg, ground
- 1 cup blackberries, pureed

Directions:

1. In the mixing bowl, combine the flour with vanilla, nutmeg and the other ingredients except the cooking spray and whisk.

2. Spray the crockpot bottom with the cooking spray.
3. Pour pancake batter in the crockpot and flatten it gently.
4. Cook the pancake for 6 0 minutes on High.
5. Then open the lid and add butter.
6. Let the pancake rest for 25 minutes.

Ricotta And Pecan Cupcakes

Ingredients:
- 4 tablespoons butter, frozen
- 2 teaspoon Ricotta cheese
- 2 tablespoons pecans, chopped
- 2 tablespoon stevia
- 2 cup almond flour
- 2 teaspoon almond extract
- 2 teaspoon ground nutmeg

Directions:
1. Mix up together the flour with almond extract and the other ingredients and stir until you obtain a dough
2. After this, transfer the dough in the freezer for 25 minutes.
3. Remove the dough from the freezer and grated it.
4. Divide the dough into muffin molds.

5. After this, arrange the cupcakes in the crockpot.
6. Close the lid and cook them on High for 4 hours.

Dessert Pancakes

Ingredients:
- 2 teaspoon baking powder
- 2 cup almond flour
- 2 egg, beaten
- 2 tablespoon butter
- 2 teaspoon olive oil
- 1/2 cup almond milk, unsweetened
- 2 teaspoon vanilla extract
- 2 teaspoon ground cinnamon

Directions:
1. Whisk the egg and combine it with the almond milk, vanilla extract, ground cinnamon, baking powder, and almond flour.
2. Add the butter and stir it until smooth.
3. Spray the slow cooker with the olive oil.
4. Pour the pancake batter into the slow cooker and cook for 2 hours on High.
5. Cut the pancake into servings and enjoy!

Lava Cake

Ingredients:

- 1/2 cup almond milk, unsweetened
- 4 tablespoons liquid stevia
- 2 oz dark chocolate
- 2 tablespoon cocoa powder
- 6 tablespoons almond flour

Directions:

1. Combine the cocoa powder and almond flour.
2. Add almond milk and liquid stevia.
3. Stir the mixture until smooth.
4. Place the batter in ramekins and place the dark chocolate in the center of the cake.
5. Cook the lava cake for 2.6 hours on High.
6. Serve the cake immediately while hot!

Almond Coffee Cream

Ingredients:

- 2 cup brewed coffee
- 1 cup coconut cream
- 2 tablespoon coconut oil
- 2 tablespoons almonds, chopped
- 2 oz dark chocolate, melted

Directions:

1. In your crockpot, mix the chocolate with coffee and the other ingredients, close the lid and cook on High for 40 minutes.
2. Divide into bowls and serve cold.

Brown Fudge Cake

Ingredients:
- 1 teaspoon of baking powder
- 2 teaspoons of fresh orange zest, grated finely
- Erythritol, as required
- 4 ramekins
- 2 tablespoons of extra-virgin olive oil
- 2 egg
- 1/2 cup of almond flour
- 1/2 cup of erythritol
- 2 tablespoon of cocoa powder

Directions:
1. Separately blend the wet and dry Ingredients: in the mixer while reserving the berries.
2. Mix both the mixtures together in a bowl until smooth.
3. Divide this batter into 4 ramekins and place them in the crockpot.

4. Cover its lid and cook for 4 hours on Low setting.
5. Once done, remove its lid of the crockpot carefully.
6. Allow them to cool and refrigerate for 2 hour.
7. Serve.

Orange Cheese Cake

Ingredients:

- zest of 1/2 orange
- 4 egg, room temp
- 1 jar Greek yogurt
- 4 raspberries
- 2 cup of water
- 1/2 cup of erythritol
- 1 teaspoon of almond flour
- 1/2 teaspoon of vanilla
- 2 tablespoons of sour cream
- 1 tablespoon of lemon Juice

Directions:

1. Separately blend the wet and dry Ingredients: in the mixer.
2. Mix both the mixtures together in a bowl until smooth.
3. Now spread the cake batter in a greased ramekin and place it in the Crockpot.
4. Cover its lid and cook for 4 hours on Low setting.

5. Once done, remove its lid of the crockpot carefully.
6. Allow it to cool and refrigerate for 2 hour.
7. Serve.

Walnut Cake

Ingredients:

- 2 tablespoons walnuts, chopped
- 4 eggs, beaten
- 1/2 cup coconut milk
- 2 egg yolks
- 2 teaspoon peanut butter
- 2 cup almond flour
- 4 tablespoons butter, softened
- 2 teaspoon almond extract
- 1 cup stevia
- 4 tablespoons Ricotta cheese

Directions:

1. In a bowl, mix the coconut milk with the flour and the other ingredients and whisk well.
2. Line the slow cooker with baking paper, pour the cake mix inside and close the lid.
3. Cook the mix for 4.6 hours on Low.
4. Cool down and serve.

Toffee Pudding

Ingredients:
- 2 pinch salt
- 6 tablespoons of brown swerve
- 2 /6 cup of unsalted butter
- 1 egg
- 1 teaspoon of vanilla extract
- 1/2 cup of sugar-free maple syrup
- 1/2 cup of boiling water
- 1/3 cup of almond flour
- 1 teaspoon of baking powder

Directions:
1. Start by blending all the Ingredients: together in a mixer.
2. Pour this mixture into 4 ramekins and place them in the Crockpot.
3. Cover its lid and cook for 4 hours on Low setting.
4. Once done, remove its lid of the crockpot carefully.

5. Allow it to cool and refrigerate for 2 hour.
6. Serve.

Soft Bacon Cookies

Ingredients:
- 4 oz bacon, chopped cooked
- 2 teaspoon olive oil
- 2 teaspoon stevia extract
- 1 cup almond flour
- 2 egg, beaten
- 4 tablespoons butter, melted

Directions:
1. Whisk the egg and mix it with the butter and olive oil.
2. Add the stevia extract and stir the mixture gently.
3. Add the almond flour and knead the dough.
4. When the dough is smooth, add the chopped bacon and knead it again.

5. Make fresh cookies by rolling the dough into fresh balls with your hands.
6. Place the cookies in the slow cooker and cook for 4 hours on Low.
7. Check if the cookies are cooked and remove them from the slow cooker.
8. Cool slightly.
9. Serve!

Raspberry Custard Trifle

Ingredients:

- 1/2 teaspoon of cinnamon, ground
- 4 tablespoons of brown swerve
- 2 tablespoons of water
- 2 cup of raspberries
- 6 eggs
- 1/3 cup of erythritol
- 2 teaspoon of vanilla extract
- 2 pinch salt

Directions:

1. Start by blending all the Ingredients: together in a mixer except raspberries, brown swerve, and water.
2. Pour this mixture into 4 ramekins and place them in the Crockpot.
3. Cover its lid and cook for 4 hours on Low setting.
4. Once done, remove its lid of the crockpot carefully.
5. Allow it to cool and refrigerate for 2 hour.

6. Meanwhile, boil brown swerve with water in a saucepan and cook until it is caramelized.
7. Garnish the custard with raspberries then pour the caramel mixture on top.
8. Serve.

Vanilla Avocado Cookies

Ingredients:
- 2 tablespoon stevia
- 2 tablespoon butter
- 1 teaspoon avocado oil
- Cooking spray
- 1 cup almond flour
- 2 avocado, peeled, pitted and mashed
- 1 teaspoon vanilla extract

Directions:
1. In the mixing bowl, mix up together flour with avocado and the other ingredients except the cooking spray and stir until you obtain a dough
2. Knead the soft but non-sticky dough.
3. Brush the crockpot bowl with cooking spray from inside.
4. Make the fresh balls from the dough and press them gently with the help of the fork.

5. Put the cookies in the crockpot and cook for 2 hour on High.

Chocolate Cheese Cake

Ingredients:
- 2 tablespoon of powdered peanut butter
- 1 teaspoon of pure vanilla extract
- 1/3 tablespoon of cocoa powder
- 2 egg
- 8oz. cream cheese softened

Directions:
1. Separately blend the wet and dry Ingredients: in the mixer while reserving the berries.
2. Mix both the mixtures together in a bowl until smooth.
3. Now spread the cake batter in a greased ramekin and place it in the Crockpot.
4. Cover its lid and cook for 3-4 hours on Low setting.
5. Once done, remove its lid of the crockpot carefully.

6. Allow it to cool and refrigerate for 2 hour.
7. Serve.

Candied Almonds

Ingredients:

- 4 tablespoons water
- 1/2 teaspoon ground cinnamon
- 2 cup almonds
- 1/2 cup granulated monk fruit sweetener

Directions:

1. Mix the sweetener and water.
2. Add the ground cinnamon and stir.
3. Place the almonds in the slow cooker.
4. Add the sweetener mix and stir.
5. Cook the almonds for 4 hours on High.
6. Cool the dessert a little.
7. Enjoy!

Avocado And Walnuts Balls

Ingredients:
- 2 tablespoon stevia
- 2 tablespoons walnuts, chopped
- 1 teaspoon vanilla extract
- 2 avocado, pitted, peeled
- 2 oz dark chocolate
- 4 tablespoons almond butter

Directions:
1. In the crockpot, mix the chocolate with almond butter and the other ingredients except the avocado.
2. Close the lid and cook on Low for 6 hours.
3. Meanwhile, place the avocado in the blender and blend until fluffy.
4. When the time is over, open the crockpot lid and transfer the walnuts mix in the mixing bowl.

5. Add blended avocado and stir until homogenous.
6. Chill the mixture in the fridge for 2 6 -25 minutes.
7. Make the fresh balls from the mixture, arrange on a platter and keep in the fridge until serving.

Maple Custard

Ingredients:
- 2 teaspoon of maple extract
- 1/2 teaspoon of salt
- 1 teaspoon of cinnamon
- 2 cup of heavy cream horizon organic
- 1 cup of almond milk
- 1/2 cup of swerve

Directions:

1. Start by blending all the Ingredients: together in a mixer.
2. Pour this mixture into a 4 oz.
3. ramekin and place it in the Crockpot.
4. Cover its lid and cook for 2 hours on Low setting.
5. Once done, remove its lid of the crockpot carefully.
6. Allow it to cool and refrigerate for 2 hour.
7. Garnish as desired.

Cream Cheese Cookies

Ingredients:

- 1/2 cup avocado oil
- 2 cup almond flour
- 2 fresh egg, beaten
- 2 teaspoon cream cheese
- 2 teaspoon almond extract
- 2 teaspoon baking soda
- 2 tablespoon apple cider vinegar
- 4   tablespoons sugar-free chocolate chips
- 1/2 cup stevia

Directions:

1. In a bowl, mix the egg with flour, cream cheese and the other ingredients and whisk.
2. Transfer the cookies mixture in the slow cooker.

3. Flatten the surface of the cookie dough with the help of the spatula.
4. Cook the chip cookies for 6 hours on Low.

Chocolate Cheesecake

Ingredients:

- 2 cup powder sweetener of your choice, Swerve (or suitable substitute)
- 2 teaspoon vanilla extract
- 1 cup sugarless dark chocolate chips
- 4 cups cream cheese
- Pinch of salt
- 4 fresh eggs

Directions:

1. In a bowl, beat together the cream cheese, sweetener, and salt.
2. Add the fresh eggs one at a time. Combine thoroughly.
3. Spread the cheesecake in a cake pan, which fits in the crock-pot you are using.
4. Melt the chocolate chips in a small pot and pour over the batter.

5. Using a knife, swirl the chocolate through the batter.
6. Pour 2 cups of water in the crock-pot and set the cake pan inside.
7. Attention: Careful the water does not exceed the level of the cake pan.
8. Cover the pot with a paper towel to absorb the water.
9. Cover, cook on high for 4 hours. Remove from the crock-pot and let it cool in the pan for 2 hour. Refrigerate.

Lime Vanilla Bites

Ingredients:

- 2 tablespoons lime juice
- 1 teaspoon baking soda
- 6 tablespoons coconut flour
- 2 fresh egg, beaten
- ¾ cup butter, softened
- 1 teaspoon vanilla extract
- 2 tablespoon stevia
- 2 teaspoon lime zest, grated

Directions:

1. Mix up together the butter with vanilla, stevia and the other ingredients until smooth.
2. Then put the mixture into 4 ramekins and flatten gently.
3. Transfer the ramekins in the slow cooker.

4. Cook the lemon bites for 2 hours on High.

Crockpot Lemon Custard

Ingredients:
- 1 cup of erythritol
- 2 cups of whipping cream or coconut cream
- Lightly sweetened whipped cream
- 1/2 cup of freshly squeezed lemon juice
- 2 tablespoon of lemon zest
- 2 teaspoon of vanilla extract

Directions:
1. Start by blending all the Ingredients: together in a mixer.
2. Pour this mixture into 4 ramekins and place them in the Crockpot.
3. Cover its lid and cook for 2 hours on Low setting.

4. Once done, remove its lid of the crockpot carefully.
5. Allow it to cool and refrigerate for 2 hour.
6. Garnish as desired.
7. Serve.

Keto Truffles

Ingredients:
- 2 tablespoons butter
- 4 tablespoon almond flour
- 2 tablespoon coconut flour
- 2 fresh egg, beaten
- 2 tablespoons cocoa powder
- 2 tablespoon Erythritol
- 2 oz dark chocolate

Directions:
1. Mix the Erythritol, butter, almond flour, and coconut flour.

2. Add the beaten egg and stir until smooth.
3. Melt the chocolate and add it to the flour mixture.
4. Knead until smooth.
5. Make small balls from the dough and coat them in the cocoa powder.
6. Place the truffles in the slow cooker and cook for 2 hours on High.
7. Cool truffles and serve!

Avocado Muffins

Ingredients:
- 4 tablespoons almond flour
- 2 tablespoon butter
- 2 teaspoons liquid stevia
- 2 teaspoon coconut flour
- 2 fresh egg, beaten
- 2 teaspoon baking powder
- 2 avocado, mashed

Directions:

1. Whisk together the egg and mashed avocado.
2. Add the baking powder and almond flour.
3. Add the butter and liquid stevia.
4. Sprinkle the mixture with the coconut flour and knead the dough.
5. Place the dough in 4 muffin molds.
6. Transfer the muffins to the slow cooker and cook for 4 hours on High.
7. Cool the cooked muffins and serve!

Vanilla Cream

Ingredients:

- 2 cup almond milk, unsweetened
- 2 teaspoon ground cinnamon
- 1 teaspoon turmeric
- 2 egg whites
- 4 tablespoons Erythritol
- 2 teaspoon vanilla extract

Directions:

1. Whisk the egg whites until soft peaks and add Erythritol.
2. Add the vanilla extract and almond milk.
3. Keep whisking the mixture for 2 minutes more.
4. Then add the ground cinnamon and turmeric.
5. Stir the mixture gently and transfer to the slow cooker.
6. Cook the cream for 2 hours on Low.
7. Transfer the cooked dessert into ramekins and enjoy!

Cayenne Mousse

Ingredients:
- ¾ teaspoon cayenne pepper
- 4 tablespoons organic almond milk
- 2 teaspoon liquid stevia
- 4 tablespoons butter, softened
- 2 oz dark chocolate, soft

- 2 cup heavy cream

Directions:
1. In the crockpot, mix the chocolate with the cream and the other ingredients and whisk well.
2. Close the lid and cook the mixture on High for 2 hour.
3. After this, open the crockpot divide the mousse into bowls and serve.

Creamy Mousse

Ingredients:
- 2 tablespoon stevia
- 2 eggs, beaten
- 1 teaspoon almond extract
- 2 cup heavy cream
- ¾ cup coconut cream
- 2 tablespoons Ricotta cheese

Directions:
1. In the mixing bowl whisk together cream with Ricotta and the other ingredients and whisk well.
2. When the liquid is smooth, pour it in the crockpot and cook for 6 hours on Low.
3. When the time is over, pour the liquid in the blender and blend until it is fluffy.
4. Then pour the mousse in the serving cups and chill for 2-4 hours in the fridge or 2 hour in the freezer.
5. Stir the mousse every 45 minutes.

Mint Cake

Ingredients:
- 1 cup of coconut milk
- 2 teaspoon butter, melted
- 2 teaspoon baking soda
- 2 cup almond flour
- 1 cup Monk fruit
- 2 teaspoon dried mint
- 2 teaspoon mint extract
- 2 teaspoon almond extract
- 2 cup almond flour

Directions:
1. Line the crockpot with baking paper.
2. In the big mixing bowl mix up together all ingredients.
3. When you get a smooth batter, pour it in the crockpot.
4. Flatten it gently and close the lid.
5. Cook the mint cake on High for 4 hours.

6. When the cake is cooked, chill it well and only then remove from the crockpot.
7. Slice it into the servings.

Leeks Soup

Ingredients:
*   1 cup heavy cream
*   2 teaspoon salt
*   2 teaspoon ground black pepper
*   1 teaspoon oregano, dried
*   4 leeks, sliced
*   4 and 1 cups of water
*   4 spring onions, chopped
*   2 teaspoon butter, soft

Directions:
1. In the slow cooker, mix the leeks with the water and the other ingredients except the cream.
2. Close the lid and cook soup for 4 hours on High.

3. When the time is over, open the lid and add heavy cream blend with an immersion blender.
4. Close the lid and cook the soup for 45 minutes more on High.
5. Divide into bowls and serve.

Whole Roasted Chicken

Ingredients:
- 2 teaspoons sweet paprika
- 2 teaspoon Cayenne pepper
- 2 teaspoon onion powder
- 2 teaspoon ground thyme
- 2 teaspoons fresh ground black pepper
- 4 Tablespoons butter, cut into cubes
- 2 whole chicken
- 4 garlic cloves
- 6 small onions
- 2 Tablespoon olive oil, for rubbing
- 2 teaspoons salt

Directions:

1. Mix all dry ingredients well.
2. Stuff the chicken belly with garlic and onions.
3. On the bottom of the crock-pot, place four balls of aluminium foil.
4. Set the chicken on top of the balls.
5. Rub it well with olive oil.
6. Cover the chicken with seasoning, drop in butter pieces.
7. Cover, cook on low for 8 hours.

Spinach Leeks Dip

Ingredients:
- 4 cups of spinach, torn
- 1/2 cup of vegetable broth
- 1/2 cup of lime juice
- 2 bunch basil, diced
- A pinch of salt and black pepper
- 2 tablespoons of avocado oil
- 2 leeks, diced
- -2 garlic cloves, minced

Directions:
1. Start by throwing all the Ingredients: into the Crockpot.
2. Cover its lid and cook for 6 hours on Low setting.
3. Once done, remove its lid of the crockpot carefully.
4. Blend this dip mixture using an immersion blender.
5. Mix well and garnish as desired.

6. Serve warm.

Mini Lamb Burgers

Ingredients:
- 25 small slices/pieces of cheddar cheese
- 25 small lettuce leaves1 cup mayonnaise
- 25 cucumber slices
- 2 lb minced lamb
- 4 garlic cloves, crushed
- 2 tsp mixed dried herbs
- 2 fresh egg, lightly beaten

Directions:
1. In a medium-sized bowl, mix together the minced lamb, garlic, dried herbs, fresh egg, salt, and pepper until combined.
2. Roll the mixture into 25 balls, and flatted with your palms to create a mini patty.
3. Drizzle some olive oil into the Crock Pot.
4. Place the lamb patties into the pot.

5. Place a slice of cheese on top of each patty.
6. Place the lid onto the pot and set the temperature to HIGH.
7. Cook for 4 hours.
8. Preheat the oven to 200 degrees Celsius on the GRILL setting.
9. Place the cheese-covered patties onto an oven tray and place into the hot oven.
10. Grill for a few minutes until the cheese is bubbling and the edges of the patties are golden.
11. Assemble the burgers by placing a patty onto a lettuce leave, then placing a dollop of mayonnaise on top, followed by a cucumber slice, fold the lettuce over so that it encases the fillings.
12. Serve on a platter!

Tomato Chili

Ingredients:
- 2 teaspoon oregano, dried
- 2 teaspoon ground black pepper
- 2 teaspoon salt
- 2 green bell pepper, chopped
- 1/2 cup vegetable stock
- 2 teaspoon chili powder
- 2 -pound tomatoes, roughly cubed
- 2 jalapeno pepper, chopped
- 2 spring onions, chopped
- 2 cup kale, chopped

Directions:
1. In the slow cooker, mix the tomatoes with the kale and the other ingredients.
2. Then close the slow cooker lid and cook on Low for 6 hours.
3. Divide into bowls and serve.

Turkey Taco Meat

Ingredients:

- 2 tablespoons soy sauce
- 4 oz. tomato sauce, low-carb and sugar-free
- 2 cup diced white onion
- 5 tablespoons Mexican-seasoning blend

Directions:

1. Grease a 4-quart slow-cooker with a non-stick cooking spray and add all of the ingredients.
2. Season with a pinch of salt and ground black pepper.
3. Cover and seal the slow-cooker with its lid, and set the cooking timer for 4 to 6 hours.
4. Allow to cook at a low heat setting.
5. Garnish with chopped green onion and serve in lettuce wraps.

Cheesy Broccoli And Leek Soup

Ingredients:

- 4 garlic cloves, finely chopped
- 2 cups vegetable or chicken stock
- 2 cup grated cheddar cheese
- 2 cup full-fat cream
- 2 large head of broccoli, cut into small pieces
- 2 large leek, sliced

Directions:

1. Drizzle some olive oil into the Crock Pot.
2. Add the broccoli, leek, garlic, stock, salt, and pepper to the pot, stir to combine.
3. Place the lid onto the pot and set the temperature to HIGH.
4. Cook for 4 hours.
5. With a hand-held stick blender, blend the soup until smooth.

6. Add the cheese and cream to the soup and stir.
7. Place the lid back onto the pot and cook on HIGH for another hour, or until the cheese has melted.
8. Serve while hot!

Keto Crock Pot Beef & Broccoli

Ingredients:
- 1/2 teaspoon red pepper flakes
- 1 teaspoon sea salt
- 2 head broccoli, chopped
- 2 red bell pepper
- 2 teaspoon sesame seeds
- 1/2 cup liquid Aminos
- 2 cup beef broth
- 4 tablespoons of Stevia
- 2 teaspoon fresh ginger, grated
- 4 garlic cloves, minced

Directions:
1. Preheat Crock Pot on LOW.
2. Slice flank steak into small chunks.
3. In Crock Pot add steak, Amino, sweetener, beef broth, ginger, garlic cloves, salt and red pepper flakes.
4. Cover and cook on LOW for 6 hours.

5. Prepare the broccoli and red peppers.
6. Chop broccoli florets and slice red pepper into large thin pieces.
7. After steak has cooked stir.
8. Add in the broccoli and pepper on top for the last hour of the cook time.
9. Sprinkle with sesame seeds for garnish and serve.

Creamy Parmesan Green Beans

Ingredients:
- 1/2 cup of parmesan, grated
- 2 teaspoon of lemon zest, grated
- Salt and black pepper- to taste
- A pinch red pepper flake
- 1 cup of heavy cream
- 2 cup of mozzarella, shredded

Directions:

1. Start by throwing all the Ingredients: into your Crockpot.
2. Cover its lid and cook for 2 hours on Low setting.
3. Once done, remove its lid and give it a stir.
4. Garnish as desired.
5. Serve warm.

Creamy Beef Mix

Ingredients:
- 2 teaspoon garam masala
- 2 teaspoon cayenne pepper
- 2 teaspoon salt
- 2 spring onions, chopped
- 1/2 cup cremini mushrooms, diced
- 2 tablespoon fresh parsley
- 25 oz beef loin, roughly cubed
- 2 cup heavy cream
- 2 teaspoon coconut oil, melted
- 2 teaspoon turmeric powder

Directions:
1. Heat up a pan with the oil over medium-high heat, add the meat, turmeric, masala and cayenne, toss, and brown for 6 minutes.
2. Then transfer meat in the slow cooker.
3. Add the rest of the ingredients and close the lid.

4. Cook beef stroganoff for 10 hours on Low.

Ginger Broccoli Stew

Ingredients:
- 2 broccoli head, florets separated
- 2 teaspoon of coriander seeds
- 2 tablespoon of olive oil
- 2 yellow fresh onion, diced
- Salt and black pepper- to taste
- A pinch red pepper, crushed
- 2 small ginger piece, diced
- 2 garlic clove, minced

Directions:
1. Start by throwing all the Ingredients: into your Crockpot.
2. Cover its lid and cook for 4 hours on Low setting.
3. Once done, remove its lid and give it a stir.

4. Garnish as desired.
5. Serve warm.

Eggplant Mushroom Soup

Ingredients:
- 2 tablespoons of white wine
- 2 tablespoon of olive oil
- 2 tablespoon of dry porcini mushrooms, soaked and drained
- 1 teaspoon of salt
- 1 teaspoon of black pepper
- 2 eggplant, peeled and diced
- 2 red fresh onion, diced
- 2 cup of creme fraiche
- 4 cups of vegetable stock
- 2 cup of spinach, chopped

Directions:
1. Start by throwing all the Ingredients: except crème Fraiche and slice mushrooms into your Crockpot.

2. Mix well and cover the Crockpot with its lid.
3. Select the Low settings for 6 hours.
4. Stir in crème Fraiche and puree the soup until smooth.
5. Garnish with sliced mushrooms.
6. Serve warm.

Hashed Plantain and Pork Browns

Ingredients:
- 5 tsp garlic powder
- 5 tsp olive oil
- 5 bay leaves
- 1/3 cup beef broth
- 6 plantains, peeled and halved
- 2 lb pork sirloin roast, fat trimmed
- 5 tsp sea salt

- 5 tsp ground cumin

Instructions:

1. In a bowl, mix together the garlic powder, pepper, salt, and cumin.

2. Rinse the pork, then pat dry with paper towels.

3. Rub the the cumin mixture all over the roast.

4. Place a heavy skillet over medium high flame and heat the olive oil.

5. Cook the pork until browned all over.

6. Drain the excess fat and collect in a clean container.

7. Transfer the pork to the slow cooker.

8. Pour the beef into the slow cooker, then add the bay leaf.

9. Cover and cook for 8 hours on low.

10.   About halfway into the slow cooking time, place a skillet over medium high flame and heat the reserved pork fat.

11.   Add the plantains and cook until browned.

12.   Using a slotted spoon, transfer the plantains to the slow cooker.

13.   Cover and allow to cook to the full 8 hours.

14.   Remove the bay leaf, then take the roast out and place on a chopping board.

15.   Set aside to cool.

16.   Take the plantains out of the slow cooker, then dice.

17.   Place in a large bowl and set aside.

18.   Shred the roast using two forks, then add to the plantain mixture.

19.   Mix well, then serve, preferably with scrambled eggs.

Asian Rice Pudding

Ingredients:

- 2 tsp minced scallions
- 2 tsp coriander
- Fish sauce, as needed
- 2 cups uncooked white rice, rinsed
- 25 cups gluten free chicken broth
- 6 cloves garlic, chopped

Instructions:

1. Combine the rice, chicken broth, and garlic in the slow cooker.

2. Cover and cook for 8 hours on low, or until rice is tender.

3. Ladle into bowls and sprinkle the scallions and coriander on top.

4. Serve with fish sauce.

Hazelnut Bread

Ingredients:

- 1/3 tsp sea salt
- 5 tsp walnut oil
- 5 cups unflavored almond milk
- 1 cup raw honey
- 1/3 cup chopped walnuts
- 2 cups hot water
- 5 tsp baking soda
- 2 1 cups hazelnut flour
- 1/3 tsp ground nutmeg
- 1/3 tsp ground cinnamon

Instructions:

1. Set the slow cooker on low heat.
2. Add about an inch of hot water.

3. Put a grilling or cake rack into the slow cooker.

4. Put the lid on and let stand.

5. Mix together the hazelnut flour, cinnamon, baking soda, nutmeg, and salt in a bowl using a whisk or wooden spoon.

6. Stir in the almond milk, then the honey.

7. Mix until just combined; do not over-mix.

8. Gently stir in the walnuts until evenly distributed in the batter.

9. Rub walnut oil all over the inside of deep casserole or soufflé dish that would fit inside the slow cooker.

10.   Pour the batter into it, then cover with aluminum foil.

11.   Place the casserole or dish inside the slow cooker, cover, and cook for 4 hours on low.

12.   Poke the center of the bread using a toothpick, and if it comes out clean then it is ready.

13.   Carefully take the casserole or dish out of the slow cooker and place on a wire rack.

14.   Take off the aluminum foil, then set aside for 30 minutes.

15.   Run a knife along the edge of the bread to loosen it from the casserole or dish.

16.   Invert onto the wire rack and set aside to cool for an additional 25 minutes.

17.   Slice, then serve.

Mexican Scrambled Fresh eggs

Ingredients:

- 1 cup chopped onion
- 2 oz canned chopped green chilies, drained
- 2 cup grated Monterrey Jack cheese
- 1 lb breakfast sausage, browned and drained
- 1 cup chopped green bell pepper

  4 fresh eggs

- Non-stick cooking spray

Instructions:

1. Grease the slow cooker with non-stick cooking spray.

2. Spread the cooked breakfast sausage on the bottom of the slow cooker in a single layer.

3. Spread the onions on top of the layer, followed by the peppers, then the chilies and cheese.

4. Beat the fresh eggs in a bowl then pour on top of everything.

5. Cover and cook for 6 hours on low.

6. Carefully remove from the slow cooker, slice and serve.

White Chocolate

Ingredients:

- 2 1 cups gluten free white chocolate chips
- 4 tsp vanilla extract
- 4 1 cups skimmed milk
- 4 1 cups non-fat evaporated milk

Instructions:

1. Combine the ingredients in the slow cooker.

2. Cover and cook for 4 hours on low or for 2 hour on high.

3. Pour into a thermos or serve immediately.

Cranberry and Orange Cider

Ingredients:

- 2 cup cranberry juice
- 1 cup orange juice
- 2 cinnamon sticks
- 2 cups apple cider
- 1/3 cup apricot nectar

Instructions:

1. Pour the ingredients into the slow cooker and stir to combine.

2. Cover and cook for 6 hours on low.

3. Remove the cinnamon sticks and serve immediately.

Pineapple Orange Tea

Ingredients:

- 1/3 cup orange juice
- 1/3 cup pineapple juice
- 1 orange, divided into segments
- 4 cups boiling water
- 4 tea bags of choice
- 5 Tbsp honey

Instructions:

1. In the slow cooker, place the tea bags.

2. Pour the boiling water on top and let steep for 6 minutes.

3. Remove the tea bags and stir in the orange and pineapple juices, honey, and orange segments.

4. Cover and cook for 2 hours on low. Serve immediately.

Wassail

Ingredients:

- 1/2 tsp allspice
- 2 cups orange juice
- 1/3 cup lemon juice
- 4 quarts apple juice or apple 1 cup water
- 1 cup coconut sugar
- 1/2 tsp ground ginger
- 1/3 cinnamon stick

cider

Instructions:

1. Combine the coconut sugar, ground ginger, cinnamon sticks and allspice in a large saucepan and place over low medium flame.

2. Stir constantly as you bring to a simmer.

3. Continue to stir until the sugar completely dissolves.

4. Stir in the apple juice or apple cider, orange juice and lemon juice until heated through.

5. Pour the mixture into the slow cooker, cover, and cook for 2 hour and 45 minutes on low.

6. Pour into a heatproof pitcher and serve warm or refrigerate and serve chilled.

Happy Day Punch

Ingredients:

- 1/2 cup coconut sugar or light brown sugar
- 2 cup cranberry juice
- 4 oz frozen lemonade concentrate, thawed
- 2 orange, unpeeled, sliced
- 1/3 quart apple juice or apple cider
- 5 cinnamon sticks, broken up
- 1 cup water
- 1 tsp whole cloves

Instructions:

1. Combine the cinnamon and cloves in a small cheesecloth and tie it up using kitchen string.

2. Pour the water and sugar into the slow cooker and stir until the sugar dissolves completely.

3. Pour in the lemonade concentrate and cranberry juice.

4. Place the cinnamon and clove bag into the mixture, cover and cook for 2 hours on low.

5. Take out the cinnamon and clove bag then add the orange slices.

6. Keep warm as you serve.

Crockpot Strawberry Dump Cake Recipe

Ingredients:

- 42 oz. Strawberry Pie Filling
- 1 cup butter melted
- 30 .26 oz. Betty Crocker Strawberry Cake Mix

Directions:

1. Spray with a non-stick cooking spray inside the crockpot.
2. Put the Strawberry Pie Filling into the crockpot's bottom and spread evenly.
3. Combine strawberry dry cake mixture with the butter in a mixing bowl.
4. Pour the cake/butter crumbled mixture into crockpot over

strawberries and spread evenly, covering the crockpot with a lid.

5. Cook for 2 hours at high, or 4 hours at low. Serve.

Sugar-Free Chocolate Molten Lava Cake

Ingredients:

- 2 whole egg
- 2 tablespoons butter melted, cooled
- 1/2 teaspoon baking powder
- 2 /8 teaspoon salt
- 4   ¾ teaspoons cocoa powder, unsweetened
- 2 tablespoons almond flour
- 6 tablespoons Swerve sweetener divided
- 1 cup hot water
- 2 -ounce chocolate chips, sugar-free
- 1/2 teaspoon vanilla liquid stevia
- 1/2 teaspoon vanilla extract
- 2 egg yolk

Directions:

:

1. Grease the slow cooker, mix the flour, baking powder, 2 tablespoons cocoa powder, almond flour, and 4 tablespoons of Swerve in a bowl.
2. In a separate bowl, stir in fresh eggs with melted butter, liquid stevia, vanilla extract, egg yolks, and eggs.
3. Mix the wet fixing to the dry ones and combine to incorporate fully.
4. Pour the mixture into the slow cooker.
5. Top the mixture with chocolate chips.
6. Mix the remaining swerve with cocoa powder and hot water in a separate bowl, and pour this mixture over chocolate chips.
7. Cook on low within 4 hours.
8. Once done, let cool and then serve.

Blueberry Lemon Custard Cake

Ingredients:

4 tablespoon lemon juice

1 teaspoon lemon zest

2 tablespoons coconut flour

2 1 egg separated

2 tablespoons fresh blueberries

1 cup light cream

2 /8 teaspoon salt

2 tablespoons Swerve sweetener

1/2 teaspoon lemon liquid stevia

Directions:

1. Put egg whites into a stand mixture and whip to achieve stiff peaks consistency.

2. Set the egg whites aside, whisk the yolks and the other ingredients apart from the blueberries.
3. Mix the egg whites into the batter to thoroughly combine, and then grease the slow cooker.
4. Put the batter into it, then top with the blueberries—Cook within 4 hours, low.
5. Let cool when not covered for 2 hour, then keep it chilled for at least 2 hours or overnight.
6. Serve the cake topped with unsweetened cream if you like.

Slow-Cooked Pumpkin Custard

Ingredients:

- 1/2 cup superfine almond flour
- 1 teaspoon vanilla extract
- 1 cup pumpkin puree
- 1/2 cup granulated stevia 2 large fresh eggs
- 2 tablespoons butter or coconut oil
- Dash sea salt
- 1 teaspoon pumpkin pie spice

Directions:

1. Grease a crockpot with butter or coconut oil and set aside. With a mixer, break the fresh eggs into a mixing bowl, and blend until incorporated and thickened.

2. Gently beat in the stevia, then add in vanilla extract and pumpkin puree.
3. Then blend in pumpkin pie spice, salt, and almond flour.
4. Once almost incorporated, stream in coconut oil, ghee, and melted butter.
5. Mix until smooth, then move the mixture into a crockpot.
6. Put a paper towel over the slow cooker to help absorb condensed moisture and prevent it from dripping on your pumpkin custard.
7. Then cover with a lid.
8. Now cook on low for 2 hours to 2 hours 46 minutes, and check the content after two hours elapse.
9. Serve the custard with whipped cream sweetened with a little stevia and a sprinkle of nutmeg if you like.

Almond Flour Mocha Fudge Cake

Ingredients:

- 6 tablespoons blanched almond flour
- 4 tablespoons sour cream
- 1/3 oz. unsweetened chocolate, melted
- 2 egg
- 2 tablespoon butter or coconut oil
- 6 tablespoons Swerve
- 2 /8 teaspoon Celtic sea salt
- 1/2 teaspoon vanilla or chocolate extract
- 4 tablespoons hot coffee
- 1/2 teaspoon baking soda

Directions:

1. Grease the crockpot with oil.

2. Then beat coconut oil and natural sweetener in a bowl until fully incorporated.
3. Beat in eggs, cream and chocolate.
4. In a bowl, sift baking soda and almond flour and add in the chocolate mixture.
5. Then beat in coffee, salt, and vanilla until well incorporated.
6. Once done, pour the batter into the cooking pot of the slow cooker.
7. Cook on low for 2 to 4 hours or until a toothpick inserted in the cake comes out clean.

Nutmeg-Infused Pumpkin Bread

Ingredients:

- 1/2 teaspoon ground nutmeg
- Dash teaspoon baking soda
- 1 teaspoon baking powder
- 2 tablespoons coconut sugar
- 8 tablespoons almond flour
- 2 tablespoons dried apple cranberries, unsweetened
- 4 tablespoons 2 00% apple juice, plain
- Olive oil cooking spray
- 0.6 oz. unsalted pecan pieces, toasted
- 1/2 tablespoon pure vanilla extract
- 2 tablespoon safflower oil
- 2 fresh egg white
- 2 tablespoons plain Greek yogurt
- 1/2 cup cooked and puréed pumpkin
- 2 /8 teaspoon sea salt
- Dash ground allspice

Directions:

1. Lightly grease a non-stick loaf pan with cooking spray.
2. Set aside. Mix cranberries and apple juice in a small saucepan, heat the mixture on high to boil.
3. Remove, then let cool for around 25 minutes.
4. Then mix nutmeg, baking soda, allspice, baking powder, salt, maple sugar flakes, and flour in a large bowl.
5. Set aside.
6. Now mix vanilla, oil, fresh egg whites, yogurt, pumpkin, and the cranberry mixture in a fresh bowl.
7. To the flour mixture, add the pecans and cranberry-pumpkin mixture and stir to incorporate fully.
8. Spoon the batter into the pan, and use a rubber spatula or back of a spoon to smooth the top.

9. Arrange a rack inside a crockpot to elevate the pan, and then put the pan on top.
10. Cook within 4 hours, high.
11. Cool it down within 25 minutes, before slicing, then serve.

Crockpot Baked Apples Recipe

Ingredients:

- 4 tsp. Cinnamon
- 2 tsp. Allspice
- 1/2 cup butter
- Five fresh Gala apples
- 1 cup Quaker Old Fashioned Oats
- 1 cup Brown Sugar

Directions:

1. Pour 1/2 cup of water at crockpot's edge.
2. Use a sharp knife to carefully core apples.
3. Mix the oats, cinnamon, brown sugar, and allspice.
4. Fill a single apple with a mixture of oats, sugar, and spice.
5. Use a butter pat to top each apple.

6. Set in crockpot carefully and put the lid on crockpot.
7. Cook for 4 4 hours or until finished.

Salty-Sweet Almond Butter and Chocolate Sauce

Ingredients:

- 2 -ounce dark chocolate
- 1 tsp sea salt
- Few drops of stevia
- 2 cup almond butter
- 2 ounces salted butter

Directions:

1. Place the almond butter, butter, dark chocolate, sea salt, and stevia to the crockpot.
2. Cook for 4 hours, high, stirring every 45 minutes to combine the butter and chocolate as they melt.
3. Serve or store in a fridge.

Coconut Squares with Blueberry Glaze

Ingredients:

- 4 ounces cream cheese
- 2 egg, lightly beaten
- 1 tsp baking powder
- 2 tsp vanilla extract
- 2 cup of frozen berries
- 2 cups desiccated coconut
- 2 -ounce butter, melted

Directions:

1. Beat the coconut, butter, cream cheese, egg, baking powder, and vanilla extract, using a wooden spoon in a bowl until combined and smooth.
2. Grease a heat-proof dish with butter. Spread the coconut mixture into the dish.

3. Defrost the blueberries in the microwave until they resemble a thick sauce.
4. Spread the blueberries over the coconut mixture.
5. Put the dish into the slow cooker, then put hot water until it reaches halfway up the dish.
6. Cook for 4 hours, high.
7. Remove the dish from the pot and leave to cool on the bench before slicing into small squares.

Chocolate and Blackberry Cheesecake Sauce

Ingredients:

- 5 ounces butter
- 4 ounces dark chocolate
- 1 cup fresh blackberries, chopped
- 2 tsp vanilla extract
- Few drops of stevia
- ¾ lb. cream cheese
- 1 cup heavy cream

Directions:

1. Place the cream cheese, cream, butter, dark chocolate, blackberries, vanilla, and stevia into the slow cooker.
2. Place the lid onto the pot and set the temperature to low.
3. Cook for 6 hours, stirring every 45 minutes to combine the butter and chocolate as it melts.
4. Serve, or store in a fridge.

Berry & Coconut Cake

Ingredients:

- 2 teaspoon baking soda
- 1/2 teaspoon salt
- 2 large egg, beaten with a fork
- 1/2 cup coconut flour
- 1/2 cup of coconut milk
- 2 Tablespoons coconut oil
- 4 cups fresh or frozen blueberries and raspberries
- 2 Tablespoon butter for greasing the crock
- 2 cup almond flour
- ¾ cup sweetener of your choice

Directions:

1. Butter the crockpot well.
2. In a bowl, whisk the egg, coconut milk, and oil together.

3. Mix the dry ingredients.
4. Slowly stir in the wet ingredients.
5. Do not over mix.
6. Pour the batter in the crockpot, spread evenly.
7. Spread the berries on top. Cover, cook on high for 2 hours.
8. Cool in the crock for 2 -2 hours.

Cocoa Pudding Cake

Ingredients:

- 1/2 cup whey protein
- 2 teaspoons baking powder
- 1/2 teaspoon salt
- 4 large eggs
- 1 cup butter, melted
- ¾ cup full-fat cream
- 2 teaspoon vanilla extract
- 2 Tablespoon butter for greasing the crockpot
- 5 cups ground almonds
- ¾ cup sweetener, Swerve
- ¾ cup cocoa powder

Directions:

1. Butter the crockpot thoroughly.
2. Whisk the dry fixing in a bowl.
3. Stir in the melted butter, eggs, cream, and vanilla.
4. Mix well. Pour the batter into the crockpot and spread evenly.

5. Cook within 21 to 4 hours, low.
6. If preferred   more like pudding, cook cake shorter; more dry cake, cook longer.
7. Cool in the crockpot for 45 minutes. Cut and serve.

Wonderful Raspberry Almond Cake

Ingredients:

- 4 large eggs
- 2 teaspoons of baking soda
- 1/2 teaspoon of salt
- 2 cup of Swerve
- 1 cup of melted coconut oil
- 2 cup of shredded coconut unsweetened
- 1/2 cup of powdered fresh egg whites
- 2 cup of fresh raspberries
- 1/2 cup of dark chocolate chips, sugar-free
- 2 cups of almond flour
- 2 teaspoon of coconut extract
- ¾ cup of almond milk

Directions:

1. Grease the slow cooker with butter.
2. Mix all the fixing in a bowl.

3. Pour the batter inside, then cook within 4 hours on low.

Scrumptious Chocolate Cocoa Cake

Ingredients:
- The zest from 2 lemons
- 2 large eggs
- Espresso and whipped cream for serving
- Toppings:
- 4 tablespoons of sweetener
- 1 a cup of boiling water
- 2 tablespoons of lemon juice
- 2 tablespoons of coconut oil 5 cups of ground almonds
- 1 cup of coconut flakes
- 6 tablespoons of your preferred sweetener
- 2 teaspoons of baking powder
- A pinch of salt

- 1 cup of coconut oil
- 1 cup of cooking cream
- 2 tablespoons of lemon juice

Directions:

1. Combine the baking powder, sweetener, coconut, and almonds in a large bowl.
2. Whisk together thoroughly.
3. In another bowl, combine the eggs, juice, coconut oil, and whisk together thoroughly.
4. Combine the wet and the dry ingredients and whisk together thoroughly.
5. Put the aluminum foil inside the bottom of the slow cooker.
6. Pour the batter into the slow cooker.
7. Mix all the topping fixing in a small bowl, and pour on top of the cake batter.

8. Cover the slow cooker with paper towels to absorb condensation, then cook within 4 hours on high.
9. Divide into bowls and serve with espresso and whipped cream.

Crockpot Carnitas Taco

Ingredients:
- 2 tablespoon green chilies, chopped
- 2 cups Monterey Jack cheese, shredded
- 2 envelop taco seasoning
- 2 cup tomatoes, diced

Directions:
1. Place the roast in the slow cooker and sprinkle with taco seasoning all over.
2. Pour the tomatoes and green chilies around the pork roast.
3. Cook on low for 8 hours or until the meat is very tender.
4. Use two forks to shred the meat.

5. Return the shredded meat back to the slow cooker and sprinkle cheese on top.
6. Cook for another 45 minutes on high or until the cheese has slightly melted.
7. Garnish with sour cream or cilantro if preferred.

Sautéed Cabbage

Ingredients:
- 1 cup veggie stock
- 2 teaspoon coriander, ground
- 1 teaspoon salt
- 1 oz white cabbage, shredded
- 1/2 cup butter
- 1 teaspoon black pepper

Directions:
1. In the slow cooker, mix the cabbage with the butter and the other ingredients.
2. Cook the meal for 6 hours on High.

Kale And Shrimp

Ingredients:

- 2 teaspoon dried dill
- 2 teaspoon turmeric powder
- 2 teaspoon curry powder
- 2 teaspoon salt
- 2 cups kale, chopped
- 2 cup of veggie stock
- 2 -pound shrimp, peeled and deveined

Directions:

1. In the slow cooker, mix the kale with shrimp and the other ingredients, toss and close the lid.
2. Cook meat for 2 hours on High.
3. Divide into bowls and serve.

Spinach And Olives Mix

Ingredients:
- 2 teaspoon ground black pepper
- 1 teaspoon salt
- 2 cup black olives, pitted and halved
- 2 teaspoon sage
- 2 teaspoon sweet paprika
- 2 cups spinach
- 2 tablespoons chives, chopped
- 6 oz Cheddar cheese, shredded
- 1 cup heavy cream

Directions:
1. In the slow cooker, mix the spinach with the chives and the other ingredients, toss and close the lid.
2. Cook for 4 .6 hours on Low and serve.

Beef Meatball Soup

Ingredients:
- 2 garlic cloves, minced
- 2 Tablespoons olive oil
- 4 cups lean ground beef
- 2 fresh egg
- 2 teaspoon dry savoury
- Salt and pepper to taste
- 2 cup beef broth + 2 cups hot water
- 2 cup sour cream
- 2 red bell pepper, diced
- 8-25 pearl onions, halved

Directions:
1. Preheat crock-pot on low.
2. Add vegetables and olive oil.
3. In a bowl, combine meat, egg, dry savoury, salt and pepper.
4. Mix well and shape into bite-size meatballs

5. In a pot, boil the broth, add the meatballs and heat for 2 minutes.
6. Add the meatballs, and broth to the crock-pot.
7. If necessary, add 1 cup hot water.
8. Cover, cook on low for 6 hours.
9. Open the lid and ladle out a small amount of liquid, cool it slightly and use to thin the sour cream.
10. Add salt and pepper, if needed, and return the cream mixture to the pot.
11. Stir gently, not to break the meatballs. Serve hot.

Slightly Addictive Pork Curry

Ingredients:
- 2 cup water
- 1 cup white wine
- 2 teaspoon turmeric
- 2 teaspoon ginger powder
- 2 teaspoon curry powder
- 1 teaspoon paprika
- Salt and pepper to taste
- 2.2 pounds pork shoulder, cubed
- 2 Tablespoon coconut oil
- 2 yellow onion, diced
- 2 garlic cloves, minced
- 2 Tablespoons tomato paste
- 2 small can coconut milk   1 fl ounces

Directions:
1. In a pan, heat 2 tablespoon olive oil.
2. Sauté the onion and garlic for 2-4 minutes.

3. Add the pork and brown it. Finish with tomato paste.
4. In the crock-pot, mix all remaining ingredients, submerge the meat in the liquid.
5. Cover, cook on low for 8 hours.

Spiced Chicken

Ingredients:
- 2 jalapeno pepper, sliced
- 2 teaspoon minced garlic
- 2 teaspoon ground cinnamon
- 1 teaspoon chili flakes
- 1/2 cup water
- 2 teaspoon olive oil
- 4 chicken thighs, boneless, skinless
- 2 teaspoon cumin, ground
- 2 teaspoon coriander, ground
- 2 teaspoon nutmeg, ground

Directions:
1. In the slow cooker, mix the chicken with cumin, coriander and the rest of the ingredients.
2. Close the lid and cook chicken for 4 .6 hours on High.
3. Divide into bowls and serve.

Dill Leeks

Ingredients:
- 1 teaspoon turmeric powder
- 2 teaspoon sweet paprika
- 2 tablespoon coconut cream
- 2 teaspoon butter
- 2 cups leeks, sliced
- 2 cup chicken stock
- 2 tablespoons fresh dill, chopped

Directions:
1. In the slow cooker, mix the beets with the stock, dill and the other ingredients.
2. Cook on Low for 4 hours and serve.

Creamy And Spicy Prawns

Ingredients:
- 1 cup coconut milk
- 2 tomato, diced
- ½-inch ginger root, grated
- 4 cloves of garlic, minced
- Salt and Pepper to taste
- 2 tablespoons coconut oil
- 2 teaspoon chili powder
- 2 tablespoon lime juice
- 1/2 cup cilantro leaves, chopped

Directions:
1. Place all ingredients in the crock pot.
2. Stir gently and season with salt and pepper to taste.
3. Close the lid and cook on high for 2 hours.
4. Serve warm.

Vegetable Lasagna

Ingredients:
- 1 teaspoon ground black pepper
- 2 cup Cheddar, grated
- 1 teaspoon chili flakes
- 2 tablespoon tomato sauce
- 2 teaspoon coconut oil
- 1 teaspoon butter
- 2 eggplant, sliced
- 2 cup kale, chopped
- 4 eggs, beaten
- 2 tablespoons keto tomato sauce

Directions:
1. Place coconut oil in the skillet and melt it.
2. Then add sliced eggplants and roast them for 2 minute from each side.
3. After this, transfer them in the bowl.
4. Toss butter in the skillet.

5. Place 2 beaten fresh egg in the skillet and stir it to get the shape of a pancake.
6. Roast the fresh egg pancake for 2 minute from each side.
7. Repeat the steps with remaining eggs.
8. Separate the eggplants into 2 parts.
9. Place 2 part of eggplants in the slow cooker.
10. You should make the eggplant layer.
11. Then add 1 cup chopped parsley and 2 fresh egg pancake.
12. Sprinkle the fresh egg pancakes with 1/2 cup of Parmesan.
   a. Then add remaining eggplants and second fresh egg pancake.
13. Sprinkle it with 1 part of remaining Parmesan and top with the last fresh egg pancake.
14. Then spread it with tomato sauce, kale and sprinkle with chili flakes and ground black pepper.

15. Add tomato sauce and top lasagna with remaining cheese.
16. Close the lid and cook lasagna for 6 hours on Low.

Pot Roast Beef Brisket

Ingredients:
- 2 Tablespoons apple cider vinegar
- 2 teaspoon dry oregano
- 2 teaspoon dry thyme
- 2 teaspoon dried rosemary
- 2 Tablespoons paprika
- 2 teaspoon Cayenne pepper
- 2 tablespoon salt
- 2 teaspoon fresh ground black pepper
- 6.6 pounds beef brisket, whole
- 2 Tablespoons olive oil

Directions:
1. In a bowl, mix dry seasoning, add olive oil, apple cider vinegar.
2. Place the meat in the crock-pot, generously coat with seasoning mix.
3. Cover, cook on low for 1 hours.
4. Remove the brisket from the liquid, place on a pan.

5. Sear it under the broiler for 2-4 minutes, watch it carefully so the meat doesn't burn.
6. Cover the meat with foil, let it rest for 2 hour. Slice and serve.

Chilli Beef Stew

Ingredients:
- 4 Tablespoons butter
- 2 teaspoon Cayenne pepper
- 2 Tablespoon Worcestershire sauce
- 2 teaspoon dry oregano
- 2 teaspoon dry thyme
- Salt and pepper to taste
- 4 pounds stewing beef, whole
- 2 cans Italian diced tomatoes
- 2 cup beef broth

Directions:
1. Add all the ingredients to the crock-pot, mix well.
2. Cover, cook on high for 6 hours.
3. Break up the beef with a fork, pull apart in the crock-pot.
4. Taste and adjust the seasoning, if needed.

5. Re-cover, cook for an additional 2 hours on low.

Beef Picadillo

Ingredients:
- 2 Anaheim peppers, seeded and chopped
  25 green olives, pitted and chopped
- 8 cloves of garlic, minced
- 1 cup olive oil
- Salt and pepper to taste
- 5 tablespoons chili powder
- 2 tablespoon dried oregano
- 2 teaspoon ground cinnamon
- 2 cup tomatoes, chopped

Directions:
1. Place all ingredients in the crock pot and stir.
2. Close the lid and cook on low for 25 hours.
3. Serve warm with veggies if desired

Beef Noodles With Broccoli & Tomato

Ingredients:
- 2 tablespoon / 24g of coconut oil
- 2 pinch of pepper
- 2 tablespoons / 30 gr of cherry tomatoes, diced
- 2 tablespoons / 30 gr of broccoli, diced
- 2 pinch of salt
- 2 teaspoons / 30 gr of olive oil

Directions:
1. Put the beef noodles in the bottom of the Slow Cooker pot
2. Cover with the diced broccoli and tomatoes
3. Sprinkle with a pinch of salt and pepper and with 2 teaspoons of extra virgin olive oil and the coconut oil
4. Set the cooking on LOW temperature,

Lemon Asparagus

Ingredients:
- juice of 2 lemon
- Zest of 2 lemon, grated
- 1 teaspoon turmeric
- 2 teaspoon rosemary, dried
- 8 oz asparagus
- 1 cup butter

Directions:
1. In your slow cooker, mix the asparagus with butter, lemon juice and the other ingredients and close the lid.
2. Cook the vegetables on Low for 6 hours. Divide between plates and serve.

Mini Lamb And Eggplant Skewers With Yogurt Dip

Ingredients:
- 2 lemon
- 2 large eggplant, cut into 1 even chunks
- ¾ cup full-fat Greek yoghurt
- 2 tbsp fresh mint leaves, finely chopped
- 2 lb minced lamb
- 2 garlic cloves, crushed
- 2 egg, lightly beaten

Directions:
1. In a medium-sized bowl, mix together the minced lamb, garlic cloves, egg, salt, pepper, and zest of one lemon.
2. Roll the lamb mixture into 1 balls.
3. Place the eggplant chunks on a damp tea towel and sprinkle them with salt and leave while you prepare the yoghurt dip in advance.

4. Mix together the yoghurt, fresh mint, and juice of the lemon in a small bowl, cover and store in the fridge until needed.
5. Rub the eggplant chunks with olive oil.
6. Take 4 skewers and "fill" them with alternating lamb mince balls and eggplant chunks, so that each skewer has 4 lamb mince balls and 4 eggplant chunks.
7. Drizzle some olive oil into the Crock Pot.
8. Lay the skewers into the Crock Pot and set the temperature at LOW.
9. Cook for 4 hours, turning once, after the 2-hour mark.

Carrots With Mushroom Sauce

Ingredients:
- Salt and black pepper, to taste
- 1/2 cup of heavy cream
- 2 scallion, diced
- 4 large carrots, spiralized with blade C
- 2 cup of whipping cream
- 2 garlic cloves, minced
- 2 tablespoon of fresh sage leaves, diced
- 2 lb. fresh mushrooms, sliced

Directions:
1. Start by throwing all the Ingredients: into your Crockpot.
2. Cover its lid and cook for 4 hours on Low setting.
3. Once done, remove its lid and give it a stir.
4. Garnish as desired.
5. Serve warm.